Table of contents

- Introduction..2

- Chapter One: Headache..4

- Chapter Two: Constipation...10

- Chapter Three: Fatigue..14

- Chapter Four: Hunger..19

- Chapter Five: Impaired brain function...20

- Chapter Six: Overheating...26

- Chapter Seven: Bad mood...31

- Conclusion...

....**39**

INTRODUCTION.

Water is an essential class of food that is needed adequately in the body system. Drinking adequate or enough water is important, as water is required to perform nearly every bodily function. Many people are unknowingly mildly dehydrated most of the time, because, one loses water regularly, when one breathes, sweats and when one digest foods.

Although there is no standard amount of water you should be drinking on a daily basis, water is universally recognized as important to human health. Initially, the consequences of lack of water in the body can be fairly mild. However, long-term dehydration can be dangerous and lead to death.

The symptoms of dehydration can be experienced by each individual differently like thirst, less-frequent urination, dry skin, fatigue, light-headedness, dizziness, confusion, dry mouth and mucous membranes, increased heart rate and breathing. In children, symptoms may include, dry mouth and tongue, no tears when crying, no wet diapers for several hours, sunken abdomen, eyes, or cheeks, listlessness, irritability and skin that does not flatten when pinched when released.

The symptoms of dehydration may resemble other medical conditions or problems, always talk with your healthcare provider for a diagnosis.

CHAPTER ONE.

HEADACHE.

Our noggins are mostly the first, the most obvious part of our bodies that signal to H2O deficiency and they do so in the form of little to severe pain. The blood vessels around our brains are very sensitive, so if you do not drink sufficient water, they may react to the change in blood volume, and may increase the likelihood of headache. A dehydration headache happens when the body is dehydrated (does not get the fluids it needs). Headache pain often appears along with other symptoms of dehydration, including dizziness, extreme thirst and dry mouth. Pain usually goes away after drinking water, resting and taking pain relief medication, that is with at home remedies. If you have signs of severe dehydration such as confusion or dizziness, get medical assistance right away. Low fluids in the body system can lead to dehydration, which causes headache. Babies, young children and older adults have a higher risk of dehydration.   Also, People with certain health conditions (such as diabetes) also have an increased risk.

What do we mean by dehydration headache and what are its symptoms?

Dehydration headache is a kind of headache that occurs as a result of low water in the body system. Pain from a dehydration headache can range from mild to severe. You may feel pain all over your head or in just one spot, such as the back, front or side. You may have a throbbing (pounding) headache, or the pain might be constant. The pain might get worse when you bend over, shake your head or move around.

Other dehydration symptoms usually occur along with headache pain. These include:

- Dizziness and confusion.

- Dark urine and less need to urinate.

- Fatigue.

- Heat or muscle cramps.

- Dry mouth.

- Passing out or fainting (syncope). This happens in severe cases of dehydration.

- Loss of appetite.

- Intense thirst (although, you may not feel thirst at all).

    Symptoms of dehydration in babies and children include fewer trips to the bathroom or fewer wet diapers, pale skin and weakness or lethargy. It's essential to get medical help immediately.

    Dehydration headaches are secondary headaches because medical practitioners only know what causes them. One probably has a dehydration headache if:

- Pain is only in your head (other types of

headaches can cause pain in the neck or shoulders).

- Headache pain goes away or gets better with water and rest.

Note:

If your headache does not get better after drinking water and resting, see your personal doctor for a checkup, another condition or illness may be causing your headache.

How to control dehydration headaches.

Most dehydration headaches get better in a few hours with at home treatments. To relieve pain from a dehydration headache, one should try headache remedies such as:

- **Fluids:** Take small sips of water. Drinking too much water too quickly can affect your stomach. You can try sucking on ice cubes if you have an upset stomach. Electrolyte drinks (sports drinks) can also replace fluids. But they usually contain high sugar, so only drink them in moderation or choose one with no added sugar.

- **Rest:** Take a break from physical activity. If you are in the heat or sun, try relaxing in a cool, shady place. Give your body time to rest.

- **Ice:** Applying a cold compress to your head can relieve pain. You can also wet a washcloth with cold water.

- **Pain relievers:** Take drugs that relieve pain but avoid some headache medicines that have caffeine. Avoid these medicines, since caffeine can make dehydration worse. You can try taking an OTC pain reliever, such as:

  - Ibuprofen or Advil.

  - Aspirin.

  - Acetaminophen or Tylenol.

Note:

People who are very dehydrated most of the time need additional care.

How to prevent dehydration headache.

The best way to stay away from dehydration headache is to take enough water. To prevent dehydration, you should ensure you do the following:

- **Drink plenty of fluids:** Always take water with you when you leave home and take sips throughout the day.

- **Hydrate before you feel thirsty:** Drink fluids throughout the day. Don't wait until you feel thirsty. If you wait until you are craving water, you are already a little dehydrated.

- **Replace lose fluids:** When you are exercising or doing physical activity, take water breaks often. During some sports like swimming, you may not notice how much you are sweating. Drinking fluid throughout the day prior to participating in a sport is also useful.

- **Watch the heat:** If you are outside on a hot day, drink extra water. Rest often and find a way to stay cool in hot weather.

- **Take a break when you need to rest:** Listen to your body. If you feel tired or dizzy, take a water break.

Note:

Chronic dehydration can lead to serious medical problems, including kidney stones and urinary tract infectious (UTIS). People who are not hydrated have a higher risk of heat exhaustion and other heat illness. Dehydration can trigger or cause a migraine headache.

Also, see your healthcare provider if; headache pain does not get better after drinking water, resting and taking over the counter pain medications, when pain comes back or tends to be more severe, when you have other symptoms like vision problems, dizziness, nausea and vomiting can be signs of a serious condition and when you have signs of severe dehydration.

In a hot climate, the body will be losing water more

rapidly if you have a fever, if you are vomiting, or if you have a diarrhea.

It is certain that one won't live long without consuming a healthy amount of water.

You may be susceptible to the effects of dehydration even sooner, depending on certain factors. Water makes up 60 percent of our bodyweight. From research, in children, water makes up to 75 percent of their bodyweight. One can't survive without water for very long, but the exact amount of time one can live on the surface of the earth without water varies, this is because certain factors contribute to our body's use of water like, environmental conditions, activity level, health, age, weight, sex and food intake.

CHAPTER TWO.

CONSTIPATION.

Does low water intake into the body system cause constipation? Yes or No? If yes, we get to know here in this chapter and if no, we get to know also in this chapter.

Yes, it cause it and this is because when there is no enough water running through the digestive system, the digestive system can show signs of struggle, which typically manifest as constipation. " Not having enough water in the gastrointestinal tract can make stool drier and difficult to pass." And the more fiber we take in, the more water we need to be drinking, as fiber requires more water in order to be properly digested. Without it, one may experience bloating and gas on top of the constipation. We should also note that water is needed for the formation of saliva, which is also necessary for overall gut function. Digestion, after all, begins in the mouth. Dehydration is one of the most common causes of chronic constipation. The food one takes in makes its way from one's stomach to the large intestine, or colon. This makes us have hard stools that are difficult to pass. There are also other causes of chronic constipation like what we eat, a long distance journey, medicines, irritable bowel syndrome and pregnancy, but majorly, dehydration cause it.

Note:

Extra or additional fluids help keep the stool soft and easy to pass, but drinking more liquids does not cure constipation. In general, for healthy-average people, 8 cups a day is a good objective. Talk to your doctor about how much water is good for you.

Besides water, other fluids that can keep you hydrated include;

- Clear soups.

- Herbal teas.

- Vegetable juices.

Fluids to avoid are;

- **Taking too much caffeinated drinks** like coffee, tea and colas which are also diuretics. But as long as you drink moderate amounts, they probably won't cause dehydration.

- **Alcohol:** it is a diuretic, which gets rid of water from your body and leads to dehydration.

The main symptoms of constipation are:

- Straining when passing stool.

- Difficulty in or painful passing stool.

- Dry or hard stool.

- Passing less stool than usual.

- Having stomach ache or cramps.

- Feeling bloated and nauseous.

How to manage and treat constipation.

- Drink two to four extra glasses of water a day.

- **Self-care:** Constipation can be managed by you at home. Self-care starts by taking an inventory of what we eat and drink and then making changes.

- Medication or supplement review by one's doctor.

- Prescription medications like lactulose, e. t. c.

- If your constipation is caused by a structural problem, like blockage in the colon, intestinal obstruction, tear in the anus or the collapse of part of the rectum into the vagina, e. t. c, surgery may be the next and best option.

Poor digestion is a common symptom experienced by those with chronic fatigue syndrome. To digest food properly one needs to drink plenty of water (but not with a meal, because it dilutes stomach acid). Drink at least half a pint of water one and half hour before you eat. The water passes through the stomach and goes straight into the intestine and within an half hour, it is then secreted back into the stomach and goes into the mucous barrier. This barrier retains the sodium bicarbonate that is required to neutralize acid as it attempts to pass through the mucus. Those that are suffering from dehydration have inefficient mucous layers.

CHAPTER THREE.

FATIGUE.

In the past, you could be fatigue for a number of reasons, so it might be hard to connect this symptom to dehydration. Still, it was said that not having enough water in the body can make you feel tired. This has to do, at least in part, with the changes in blood volume that result from water shortages. So, if you are feeling the slump, having a glass of water might be a better first step than taking a caffeinated drink, which could further dehydrate you. Water is essential for carrying nutrients to our body's cells and taking away waste products. Roughly 50% to 60% of our body weight is water, yet we constantly lose water through sweat, urine and breathing. Consuming a sufficient amount of fluids in beverages and water-filled food such as fruits, vegetables and soup will help replenish the water our body lose throughout the day and can help us maintain our energy.

Caffeine occurs naturally in coffee, tea, cocoa and chocolate and is also added to some popular beverages. For some people, a cup of coffee or a can of cola is all they need to get a little energy boost. It is known from research that drinking beverages with caffeine does not cause excess fluid loss or dehydration, so these drinks can be enjoyed in moderation.

When we suffer from dehydration symptoms of chronic fatigue syndrome, learning how to cleanse and re-hydrate our body will improve our physical energy as well as reduce brain fog, headaches, skin problems, joint and muscle pain, poor digestion e .t .c .

Nearly all body functions are about fluid balance and even small changes in fluid balance can affect our performance and our daily life. If this fluid is not replaced, blood volume can drop.

As a result, the heart has to work harder in order to supply the skin and muscles with oxygen and nutrients.

As dehydration progresses, the body redirects blood to the working muscles and away from the skin, impairing your body's ability to diffuse heat. The increase in internal heat then results in muscle cramps, light-headedness and fatigue.

Many chronic fatigue syndrome sufferers report frequent headaches. Headaches are a consequence of physical and mental stress which can result from not being properly hydrated. Headaches caused through poor hydration are a condition shared by many sufferers of chronic fatigue. If you have chronic fatigue syndrome, the lack of fluids in your system can be very detrimental to decision making and to your health. When the brain suffers from poor hydration, mental fogginess, poor short term memory, dizziness, severe headaches and poor balance occurs or results.

Those with chronic fatigue syndrome often report skin problems. Our body is mostly water, so we need to replenish and maintain an optimum fluid level. Water helps flush out toxins in the body and helps to keep skin supple and healthy.

Water is the skin's own moisturizer and just as the rest of our body requires hydration and nutrients, so does our skin. When our skin suffers the effects of dehydration, skin problems occur. If one has chronic fatigue syndrome and skin problems, one may be suffering from dehydration.

The pain and swelling of the joint that is so often associated with chronic fatigue syndrome can also be as a result of joint dehydration. The cartilage that protects the surface of our bones at the joints is made up of a lot of water.

As the immune system attempts to deal with bacteria and viruses, poisons and toxins enter the lymph system to be disposed off from the body. Good circulation assists with this process, but if you have chronic fatigue syndrome, pain often prevents you from doing or having enough exercise. When we drink sufficient water, our body dilutes these toxins and our kidneys, more effectively flush out the poisons in our body. You are likely to feel worst before you feel better. You may find massage helpful.

Water is a natural diuretic and helps prevent one from feeling hungry. If you drink at least four pints of water daily, you will find out that you can more easily distinguish between real hunger and thirst. The net result of this is that you will have fewer cravings and find it easier to control your weight.

Dehydration can result in the body producing excess histamine which can trigger or lead to allergies.

How to get hydrated.

1. **Drinking sufficient water:** This makes blood flow without restriction in the body system and the toxins can be flushed out of your tissues and into your blood stream. When you are in a state of dehydration, your urine becomes dark in color. But when your liver and kidneys are processing the toxic waste and you are well hydrated, your urine becomes clear.

2. **Hydration therapy:** This simply means increasing your intake of fresh clean water to avoid dehydration. This is so essential for chronic fatigue syndrome

sufferers.

3. Adult should drink a minimum of four pints of water for optimum efficiency. And minimum of eight large glasses of pure water a day will help to improve the ravages of chronic fatigue syndrome.

> Lastly, with your re-hydration regimen, increase slowly over a few weeks to about 5 or 6 pints per day (providing you don't have kidney\renal problems) of non-carbonated water, either bottled or filtered. You will find yourself going to the bathroom more often, but it does pay you as your chronic fatigue syndrome symptoms will be less severe.

CHAPTER FOUR.

HUNGER.

Can dehydration make one feel hungry? Yes it will, but this will be explained in detail in this chapter.

Dehydration can make you feel hungry before you even know that you are thirsty. This is because both signals come from just one part of the brain, the hypothalamus and wires can get crossed. The result might be unnecessary snacking, so it's worth drinking water before eating.

Proper hydration is essential to one's survival. Our body need to consume a significant amount of water each day to function properly. This is because we constantly excrete water through sweat and urination, so our body need to regain lost fluids.

One won't live long without consuming a healthy amount of water.

People who embark on hunger strikes without food but access to water should not drink less than 1.7liters of water a day to maintain their fluid levels and prevent too much hunger because it can lead lead to death which may be early or long, but most time early.

Generally, food consumption as a result of hunger or being hungry due to being hydrated contributes to twenty (20) percent (%) of your total water intake per day. Some people tend to get even more water from their food, especially if they eat a significant amount of fruits and vegetables, which contain a high amount of water.

Note:

When one wakes up in the morning, one should drink a minimum of 2-ounce glasses of water and maximum of 3-ounce glasses as this can serve as a way of staying hydrated and preventing hunger quickly.

CHAPTER FIVE.

IMPAIRED BRAIN FUNCTION.

Drinking enough water can help in solving the problem of impaired brain function.

A 2 to 4 percent decrease in your body mass due to dehydration can make your brain off balance. It was found out that mild dehydration produce a significant increase in minor driving errors during a long drive. It should be noted that the body requires water to produce hormones and other neurotransmitters, so it is easily denoted from this that dehydration causes mood disturbances.

A 2% decrease in brain hydration can result in short-term memory loss which can lead to having trouble with mathematics computations. Prolonged dehydration causes brain cells to decrease in size and mass, a condition common to many elderly ones or people who have been dehydrated for years. Lack of mental clarity, sometimes referred to as "brain fog".

 If you are finding it hard to come with answers to easy questions, or you just can't shake the fog that has enveloped your mind, it might be as a result of being dehydrated. It was made known from research that there is a close link between drinking water and the brain function. Approximately 65% of your body is composed of water. Nearly every body function you have depend on water, but how much do you really need? According to research, average adult loses more than 70 ounces of water every day through sweating, breathing and releasing wastes.

 Researches show that you only need to be 1% dehydrated to experience a 5% decrease in cognitive function.

Mental symptoms of dehydration can include:

- Depression.

- Afternoon fatigue.

- Sleep issues.

- Loss of concentration.

- Lack of mental clarity, sometimes referred to as "brain fog".

The brain itself is made up of approximately 85% water. Water gives the brain energy to function including thought and memory processes. Water is also needed for the production of hormones and neurotransmitters in the brain. Since the brain cannot store water and you are constantly losing water through perspiration and other body functions, it is essential that you continuously hydrate. You will be able to think faster, focus more clearly and experience greater clarity when your brain is functioning on a full reserve of water.

5 Tips to stay hydrated are:

1. Make sure you drink a glass of water before exercising and sip during exercise.

2. Ensure you drink a glass of water before each meal.

3. Avoid alcohol while flying and drink water instead.

4. Drink water throughout the day even if you are indoors and in the air conditioning.

5. Eat your water by munching on water filled fruits and vegetables (watermelon, cucumbers).

Note:

Dehydration does not only impair people physically, but can also lead to cognitive decline or drawback.

According to the recent study, just a couple of hours of vigorous activity in the heat without drinking fluids or eating can greatly affect concentration.

Maintaining focus in long meetings, driving a car, or having a monotonous job in a hot factory requires attention.

However, in the face of being dehydrated, these abilities decline and diminished cognition can cause harm to the body.

Although researchers only examined the studies that involved between 1 and 6 percent loss of body mass due to dehydration. It was discovered that most severe impairments occurred starting at 2 percent and this drop in water weight can occur quickly.

Both the elderly and young children need to have their hydration closely monitored. Older persons are at a greater risk of dehydration due to improper ability to sense thirst, combined with a reduced ability to concentrate urine, losing more fluid.

On the other hand, younger children and infants are at a higher risk because they have a lower total body weight and a higher concentration of water. They also turn over electrolytes and water faster, so they lose water more quickly than adults.

Note:

An infant's total body water is about 70-to-75 percent. It is about 65 percent in children and 60 percent in adults.

Adequate hydration is essential for normal brain function and dehydration induces cognitive deterioration.

Mild levels of dehydration alter mood and cognitive function and reduce concentration, alertness and short- term memory in children and young adults. In the elderly. Making older people more vulnerable to body fluid imbalance and increasing their susceptibility to cognitive decline.

Furthermore, plasma hypertonicity, a marker of dehydration, increases the risk of ischemic stroke in hospitalized patients and nay precipitate cerebral ischemic events in susceptible elderly ones.

The mechanism responsible for these effects have not been clearly elucidated. Dehydration leads to reduction in brain volume and changes in neural activity in brain areas involved in fluid homeostasis, but little is known about the factors responsible for the alteration in cognition. One possibility is that dehydration disrupts critical cerebrovascular homeostatic mechanisms, such as the increase in cerebral blood flow (CBF) induced by neural activity or by endothelial cells, that assure that the brain receives a supply of oxygen and glucose well matched to the energy it needs.

In support of this possibility, alterations in cerebrovascular regulation are often associated with cognitive malfunction.

Furthermore, vasopressin (AVP), the plasma level of which increases with dehydration, is involved in the cerebrovascular dysfunction induced by administration of slow press or doses of angiotensin II (ANGII). The effect is due to AVP-mediated expression of the potent vasoactive peptide endothelin-1 (ET-1) in cerebral blood vessels, which, in turn, is responsible for the cerebrovascular alterations.

Therefore, in this study, we sought to determine whether dehydration affects the mechanisms regulating the cerebral microcirculation.

The effect depends on AVP-mediated oxidative stress and induction of ET-1 in cerebral blood vessels. The findings provide the first evidence to date that dehydration alters critical regulatory mechanisms of the cerebral circulation, which may reduce vascular reserves and contribute to the associated cognitive dysfunction and increased stroke risk.

CHAPTER SIX.

OVERHEATING.

Hydration helps to maintain a comfortable body temperature, which is why dehydration can make you feel overheated, especially in hot environments. If you are feeling the heat, you can try raising a glass before you lower the thermostat, because the problem may simply be that you need more coolant. Dehydration and heat stroke are two very common heat-related diseases that can be life-threatening if left untreated. Too much heat can cause health problems and can affect performance. Water is essential for body-temperature regulation, so lack of water causes an inability to keep one cool. Lack of water causes overheating because one's body loses its ability to regulate temperature properly as one's blood becomes more concentrated. Less blood flow takes away your body's normal means of losing heat-sweating, dilating blood vessels so the heat moves to the surface rather than staying deep inside your body. Dehydration can lead to hyperthermia and a fever-like symptoms e . g chills because over-heating can alter your body's normal temperature. Too much overheating is an urgent red flag and if noticed, stop exercising immediately to take an ice bath and hydrate.

If a person becomes dehydrated and cannot sweat enough to cool his or her body, his or her internal temperature may rise to dangerously high levels.

The body water has an important role as a thermoregulator, regulating the overall body temperature by helping dissipate heat. If the body becomes too hot, water is lost through sweat and the evaporation of this sweat from the skin surface removes heat from the body. Thereby, causing heat strokes.

Our bodies make a tremendous amount of internal heat and we normally cool ourselves by sweating and radiating heat through the skin. However, in certain circumstances, such as extreme heat, high humidity, or vigorous activity in the hot sun, this cooling system may begin to fail.

Symptoms of heat stroke include:

- Headache.

- Dizziness.

- Disorientation and confusion.

- Sluggishness or fatigue.

- Seizure.

- A high body temperature.

- Loss of consciousness.

- Rapid heartbeat.

- Hallucinations.

- Nausea.

- Blurred vision.

- Irritability or mood swing.

- Lack of coordination.

- Organ failure.

- Death, which is the final stage of all problems caused to the body.

Treatments for heat stroke are:

- First, get the person to a shaded area.

- Remove clothing and gently apply cool water to the skin followed by fanning to stimulate sweating.

- Apply ice packs to the groin and armpits.

- Have the person lie down in a cool area with their feet slightly elevated.

- Cool the person rapidly however you can.

Note:

Always make water available as much as you can to save the life of a person with heat stroke, it's essential to make provision for it quickly.

Heat stroke can be prevented through the following ways:

There are precautions that can protect you against the adverse or side effects of heat stroke which include the following:

- ✓ Drink plenty of fluids during outdoor activities, especially on hot days. Water and sport drinks are the drinks of choice. Avoid caffeinated tea, coffee, soda and alcohol, as these can lead to dehydration.

- ✓ Protect yourself from the sun by wearing a hat, sunglasses and using an umbrella.

- ✓ Wear lightweight, tightly woven, loose-fitting clothing in light colors.

- ✓ Schedule vigorous activity and sports for cooler times of the day.

- ✓ Increase time spent outdoors gradually to get your body used to the heat.

- ✓ During outdoor activities, take drink breaks often and mist yourself with a spray bottle to avoid becoming overheated.

- ✓ Spend as much time indoors as possible on very hot and humid days.

- ✓ Never leave children in closed cars on warm or sunny days.

Note:

If you live in a hot climate and have a chronic condition, talk to your doctor or your healthcare provider on extra precautions you can take to protect yourself against heat stroke and all form of heat related problems which can be caused from overheating. Overheating also known as hyperthermia is the opposite of hypothermia and it occurs when the body's heat regulation system becomes overwhelmed by outside factors, leading to a rise in one's internal temperature. Hyperthermia is considered separate from conditions where internal body sources, such as infection, heat-regulating problems and adverse drug reactions overdoses cause a raised body temperature.

Note:

In humans, core body temperature ranges from 93.9◦F to 97.5◦F during the day, or 37.5◦C to 39.5◦C. In contrast, people with some level of hyperthermia have a body temperature of more than 100.4◦F (38.6◦C).

Fast facts on hyperthermia:

- If a person's body temperature is more than 104◦F (40◦C), is defined as severe hyperthermia.

- One of the more serious stages of hyperthermia is heat exhaustion.

- Any activity that involves exercise in warm, humid, environments increases the risk of this condition.

Note:

The above mentioned are just by the way i.e not the main point we want to discuss here but we just digress a bit to know more on heat stroke as it is one of the effects of overheating.

CHAPTER SEVEN.

BAD MOOD.

Not being properly hydrated can affect your mood, too. It is noted that the body requires water to produce hormones and other neurotransmitters, so it is well known that dehydration causes mood disturbances.

Treatment for dehydration include:

If dehydration is early caught, dehydration can often be treated at home under a healthcare provider's guidance. In children, directions for giving food and fluids will be different according to the cause of the dehydration, so it is important to talk with your child's doctor or medical practitioner.

In cases of mild dehydration, simple rehydration is recommended by drinking fluids.

For moderate dehydration, intravenous (IV) fluids may be needed. If caught early enough, simple rehydration may be effective. Cases of serious dehydration should be treated as a medical emergency and hospitalization, along with intravenous fluids. Immediate action should be taken. It can lead to depression and anxiety and from there can lead to death. Though it would be so simplistic to say that dehydration is a direct cause for all types of depression, dehydration and depression are casually connected in many ways. In fact, one resulting symptom of chronic dehydration actually results to be depression.

Dehydration causes depression in at least three ways:

1. Dehydration saps your brain's energy. Dehydration impedes energy production in our brain. Many of our brain's functions require this type of energy become inefficient and can even shut down. The last is mood

disorders that result from this type of malfunction can be categorized with depression. Social stresses such as anxiety, fear, insecurity, ongoing emotional problems, e. t. c, including depression can be tied to not consuming enough water to the point that your brain's tissue is affected.

2. Dehydration impedes your brain's serotonin production. Depression is frequently related to a decreased level of serotonin, which is a critical neurotransmitter that heavily affects your mood. Serotonin is created from the amino acid tryptophan. Dehydration can also negatively impact amino acids, resulting in feelings of dejection, inadequacy, anxiety, irritability e .t .c .

3. Dehydration increases stress in one's body. Stress is one of the most prominent contributing factors to depression, along with a sense of powerlessness and inability to cope with stressors.

    Dehydration is the number one cause of stress in our body. In fact, dehydration and stress are interconnected. When you are stressed, your adrenal glands produce extra cortisol, the stress hormone and under chronic stress, your adrenal glands can become exhausted and resulting in lower electrolyte levels.

Drinking sufficient water can help reduce the negative psychological and physiological impacts of stress.

Dehydration rarely causes anxiety as a cause by itself, but not drinking adequate water puts you at risk for increased anxiety symptoms now, and possibly the development of higher anxiety levels in the future. In short, dehydration causes stress and when your body is stressed, you experience depression and anxiety as a result. Therefore, you must ensure you are drinking adequate water daily, especially if you are naturally anxiety-prone.

Water has been shown to have natural claiming properties, likely as a result of addressing dehydration's effects on the body and brain. Drinking enough water is an important step in managing anxiety. Even if you are not experiencing anxiety, drinking sufficient water can create feelings of relaxation. Panic attacks typically have physical triggers and one of those triggers is dehydration. Once dehydration occurs, if one is prone to panic attacks, one can easily begin to panic, even to the point of feeling like one is dying.

When dehydrated, you expose yourself to many symptoms that trigger panic attacks, such as

- Increased heart rate.

- Headaches.

- Muscle fatigue and weakness.

- Feeling faint\lightheaded.

While keeping yourself hydrated may not stop the panic attacks, they may become less frequent, or at least some of the triggers may be diminished.

Keeping yourself adequately hydrated is not an overall cure for depression or anxiety. You will definitely want to seek the assistance of a mental health professional.

But getting in the habit of drinking enough water daily will definitely help alleviate many of the causes and symptoms of mood volatility. Make it an important part of your daily activities or tasks.

How dehydration can be prevented are:

- ✓ Make sure you drink plenty of fluids, especially when working or playing in the sun.

- ✓ Make sure you are taking in more fluid than you are losing.

- ✓ Try to schedule physical outdoor activities for the cooler parts of the day.

- ✓ Drink appropriate sports drinks to help maintain electrolyte balance.

- ✓ For infants and young children, solutions such as Pedialyte will help maintain electrolyte balance during illness or heat exposure.

Fruits and vegetables with the highest amount of water are:

- Cabbage.

- Cantaloupe.

- Celery.

- Lettuce.

- Strawberries.

- Watermelon.

Other foods that contain a high amount of water include:

- Chicken breast.

- Cottage cheese.

- Pasta.

- Salmon.

- Shrimp.

- Yogurt.

Note:

Consuming foods high in water will help prevent dehydration. However, food alone is not likely to provide an adequate amount of water to sustain you for long period of time.

Adults may just need to drink water to rehydrate. Small children may require a drink that includes sodium in addition to water to replenish the body appropriately. Children may need to take this solution in very small amounts at first.

If one is severely hydrated, intravenous administration of water and salt may be necessary.

The top seven benefits of drinking adequate water include:

1. Drinking adequate water helps maximize physical performance especially during intense exercise or high heat. If you exercise intensely and sweat, staying hydrated can help you perform at your absolute best.

2. It can help prevent and treat headache, as headache is one of the most common symptoms of dehydration.

3. Your brain is strongly influenced by your hydration status. Fluid loss of 1.5 percent in young women after exercise impair both mood and concentration, it also adds to frequency of headaches. 1.6 percent fluid loss in young men is detrimental to working memory and increased feelings of anxiety and fatigue.

4. Taking adequate water can help relieve constipation, Increasing fluid intake is often recommended as a part of the treatment protocol. Mineral water may be a particular beneficial beverage for those with constipation.

5. Drinking adequate water can help treat kidney stones. Higher fluid intake increases the volume of urine passing through the kidneys. This

dilutes the concentration of minerals, so they are less likely to crystallize and form clumps.

6. Water can help prevent hangovers which is the unpleasant symptoms experienced after drinking alcohol. Alcohol is a diuretic, so it makes you lose more water than you take in. The best ways to reduce hangovers are to drink a glass of water between drinks and have at least one big glass of water before going to bed.

7. Lastly, water can aid weight loss. Drinking plenty water can help one lose weight. This is because water can increase one's satiety and boost our metabolic rate.

Note:

Drinking of eight glasses of water a day help keep the body healthy, also water is needed to enable the brain cells function properly, to avoid cognitive problems.

Dehydration can be a serious heat-related disease.

Occasionally, dehydration can be caused by medicines, such as diuretics. These deplete body fluids and electrolytes. Thus, we should treat dehydration as soon as possible.

Humans are mostly water. We are more than 60 percent water when we were given birth to. Water is crucial to our survival and function. Despite this, drinking water and staying hydrated is more important than many people realize.

Hydration is important because water has a variety number of important roles in the body.

Water helps to:

- Balance your electrolytes.

- Cushion your joints.

- Help nutrients and oxygen reach your cells.

- Protect your organs.

- Promote healthy cardiovascular health.

- Remove bacteria from your bladder.

- Remove waste from your body.

- Regulate your body temperature.

Alternatives to water are

1. Club soda

2. Tonic water.

3. Seltzer water.

4. Flavored waters like vitamin water or life water.

5. Sparkling water.

Note: Products like tonic water and flavored water tend to contain additional ingredients.

How much water should one be drinking?

One's ideal daily water intake depends on such person's gender, weight, stress level, climate, exercise levels, e. t. c.

You should make sure you ramp up your fluid intake accordingly, if one or more of the following situations occur:

1. Chronic health conditions.

2. Pregnant/breastfeeding mothers.

3. sIllness with fever, diarrhea, vomiting.

4. Engaging in long, intense workout sessions.

Note:

You can verify how hydrated you are based on the

color of your urine. If you are adequately hydrated, your urine will give a very clear\pale yellow color, but if you are dehydrated, your urine will show a dark yellow, tan or an unclear color. If it is a dark yellow color and of a thick\syrupy consistency, that means you are very dehydrated. Drink some water.

Note:

Increasing water intake in our body system has beneficial effects to our body system, especially sleep\wake feelings, whereas decreasing water intake in our body system has detrimental effects in our body system on HIGH's mood. These harmful effects in HIGH were observed in some sleep\wake moods as well as calmness, satisfaction and positive emotions.

Lastly, always have it at the back of your mind that getting hydrated by drinking adequate water or fluids that are beneficial, fluids without caffeine plays or is an important role in solving or treating yourself when you are dehydrated.

www.ingramcontent.com/pod-product-compliance
Lightning Source LLC
Chambersburg PA
CBHW070054260726
48658CB00002B/879